Competency Based Logbook for

2nd Professional MBBS—Microbiology

Competency Based Logbook for
2nd Professional MBBS—Microbiology

As per the Competency Based Medical Education Curriculum (NMC)

Saumya Singh MBBS MD
Professor and Head, Department of Microbiology
Curriculum Incharge, United Institute of Medical Sciences
Prayagraj, Uttar Pradesh, India

Aditya Pratap Singh MBBS MS ACME Fellow
Professor and Head, Department of Anatomy
MEU Coordinator, United Institute of Medical Sciences
Prayagraj, Uttar Pradesh, India

JAYPEE

JAYPEE BROTHERS MEDICAL PUBLISHERS
The Health Sciences Publisher
New Delhi | London

JAYPEE **Jaypee Brothers Medical Publishers (P) Ltd**

Headquarters
Jaypee Brothers Medical Publishers (P) Ltd
EMCA House, 23/23-B
Ansari Road, Daryaganj
New Delhi 110 002, India
Landline: +91-11-23272143, +91-11-23272703
+91-11-23282021, +91-11-23245672
Email: jaypee@jaypeebrothers.com

Corporate Office
Jaypee Brothers Medical Publishers (P) Ltd
4838/24, Ansari Road, Daryaganj
New Delhi 110 002, India
Phone: +91-11-43574357
Fax: +91-11-43574314
Email: jaypee@jaypeebrothers.com

Overseas Office
J.P. Medical Ltd
83 Victoria Street, London
SW1H 0HW (UK)
Phone: +44 20 3170 8910
Fax: +44 (0)20 3008 6180
Email: info@jpmedpub.com

Website: www.jaypeebrothers.com
Website: www.jaypeedigital.com

Inquiries for bulk sales may be solicited at: jaypee@jaypeebrothers.com

Competency Based Logbook for 2nd Professional MBBS—Microbiology

First Edition: 2023

ISBN: 978-93-5696-227-9

Printed in India

Student's Profile

ROLL NO...

PHOTO

UNIVERSITY REG. NO..

DATE OF JOINING..

MODE OF ADMISSION...

NAME...

FATHER'S NAME...

DOB...

E-MAIL ID...

MOBILE NO..

ADDRESS (PRESENT) ....

....

....

(PERMANENT) ....

....

....

(STUDENT'S SIGNATURE)

Certificate

This is to certify that Mr/Ms ....

Roll No..., University Reg. No...

admitted in the year..................... in the .... Medical College,

.... has satisfactorily attended/completed

all the assignments/requirements mentioned in this logbook for second year MBBS course

in the subject of Microbiology/AETCOM during the period from .... to ....

She/He is/is not eligible to appear for the summative (University) assessment as on the date

given below.

Date: ....

Place: ....

(Professor and Head)

Department of Microbiology

.... Medical College

Certificate

This is to certify that Mr/Ms ....

Roll No..., University Reg. No..

admitted in the year...................... in the .... Medical College,

.... has satisfactorily attended/completed

all the assignments/requirements mentioned in this logbook for second year MBBS course

in the subject of Microbiology/AETCOM during the period from .... to ....

She/He is/is not eligible to appear for the summative (University) assessment as on the date

given below.

Date: ....

Place: ....

(Professor and Head)
Department of Microbiology
.... Medical College

Index

AETCOM: Competencies for IMG-2018 as per guidelines of National Medical Commission (NMC) of INDIA.

Instructions

1. This logbook is prepared as per the guidelines of NMC for implementation of Competency based curriculum for Phase II MBBS students in the subject of Microbiology.
2. Students are instructed to keep their logbook entries up to date.
3. Students are expected to write reflections of activities related to self-directed learning (SDL), pandemic management and AETCOM.
4. Reflections should be structured using the following guiding questions:
   a. What happened? (What did you learn from this experience?)
   b. So what? (What are the applications of this learning?)
   c. What next? (What knowledge or skills do you need to develop so that you can handle this type of situation?)
5. The logbook assessment will be based on multiple factors like:
   a. Attendance
   b. Active participation in the sessions
   c. Timely completions
   d. Quality of write up of reflections
   e. Overall presentation.

Explanation of Each Column in the Logbook Table*

Number of the Competency

The Number of the Competency addressed includes the subject initial and number (from Vol. I, II, or III of the UG Curriculum) e.g., MI 2.3

Name of Activity

Name of activity, e.g., Seminar on Liver or Group discussion or Session 1 of CPR (if the institution has numbered each activity, the number may be entered)

Date

The activity gets completed

Attempt at Activity by Learner

Indicate if:

- First attempt (or) only attempt
- Repeat (R) of a previously done activity
- Remedial activity (Re) based on the determination by the faculty

Rating

Use one of three grades:

1. Below expectations (B)
2. Meets expectations (M)
3. Exceeds expectations (E)

Decision of Faculty

- C: Activity is completed, therefore closed and can be certified, if needed.
- R: Activity needs to be repeated without any further intervention.
- Re: Activity needs remedial action (usually done after repetition did not lead to satisfactory completion).

Initial (Signature) of Faculty

Initial (signature) of faculty indicating the completion or other determination.

Initial (Signature) of the Learner

Initial (signature) of the learner if feedback has been received.

* Competency tables and its contents have been designed as per the guidelines given in NMC logbook module. Kindly refer it for further clarification. Link – www.nmc.org.in

Introduction

Learning from patients is an integral part of health professions training. Exposure to clinical content in the para-clinical phase of learning provides a clinical context and relevance to applied sciences learning. It also facilitates early involvement in the healthcare environment that serves as motivation and reference point for students, leading to their professional growth and development. Students will be able to learn the basic and clinical sciences by means of rich integrating learning activities, be these early clinical contact, clinical skills, communication skills or task-based learning sessions.

Objectives

- Help students recognize the relevance of Microbiology in diagnosis, patient care and treatment.
- Provide a context that will enhance learning and relating to the experience of patients.
- Provide an opportunity for observing basic skills in interviewing patients and doctor–patient communication.
- Recognize attitude, ethics and professionalism as integral part of the doctor–patient relationship.
- Understand the sociocultural context of disease through the study of humanities.

Section 1

Competency Assessment

Skill Competencies of Microbiology

S. No.	Topic	Competency addressed	Name of the activity	Date completed dd-mm-yyyy	Attempt at activity First only (F) Repeat (R) Remedial (Re)	Rating Below (B) expectations Exceeds (E) expectations	Decision of faculty Completed (C) Repeat (R) Remedial (Re)	Faculty initials	Feedback received Initial of learner
1.	CVS and blood	Identify the microbial agents causing rheumatic heart disease and infective endocarditis. MI 2.3							
2.	CVS and blood	Identify the causative agent of malaria and filariasis. MI 2.6							
3.	Gastrointestinal and hepatobiliary system	Identify the common etiologic agents of diarrhea and dysentery. MI 3.2							
4.	Gastrointestinal and hepatobiliary system	Identify the different modalities for diagnosis of enteric fever. Choose the appropriate test related to the duration of illness. MI 3.4							
5.	Central nervous system infections	Identify the microbial agents causing meningitis. MI 5.3							
6.	Zoonotic diseases and miscellaneous	Demonstrate the appropriate method of collection of samples in the performance of laboratory tests in the detection of microbial agents causing infectious diseases. MI 8.10							

S. No.	Topic	Competency addressed	Name of the activity	Date completed dd-mm-yyyy	Attempt at activity First only (F) Repeat (R) Remedial (Re)	Rating Below (B) expectations Exceeds (E) expectations	Decision of faculty Completed (C) Repeat (R) Remedial (Re)	Faculty initials	Feedback received Initial of learner
7.	Zoonotic diseases and miscellaneous	Choose and interpret the results of the laboratory tests used in diagnosis of the infectious diseases. MI 8.15							
8.									
9.									
10.									
11									

Integrated Topics

S. No.	Competency addressed	Name of the activity	Date completed dd-mm-yyyy	Attempt at activity First only (F) Repeat (R) Remedial (Re)	Rating Below (B) expectations Exceeds (E) expectations	Decision of faculty Completed (C) Repeat (R) Remedial (Re)	Faculty initials	Feedback received Initial of learner
1.	Identify *Candida* species in fungal scrapings and KOH mount. DR 7.2							
2.	Identify spirochete in a dark ground microscopy. DR 10.2							
3.	Identify *Staphylococcus* on a Gram stain. DR 15.2							
4.	Assist and demonstrate the proper technique in collecting specimen for blood culture. IM 1.22							
5.	Perform and interpret a sputum Gram stain and AFB. IM 3.14, 4.13, 4.14, 6.14, PE 34.11, CT 1.10							
6.	Perform and interpret a malarial smear. IM 4.15							
7.	Assist in the collection of blood, wound and various other specimen cultures. IM 4.19, 25.9							
8.	Interpret a PPD (Mantoux). IM 4.20, PE 34.7, CT 1.7							
9.	Identify common parasitic causes of diarrhea under the microscope in a stool specimen. IM 16.9							
10.	Identify *Vibrio cholerae* in a hanging drop specimen. IM 16.10							
11.	Perform and interpret stool examination including hanging drop. PE 24.12							

Ethics and Communication Skills in Microbiology

S. No.	Competency addressed	Name of the activity	Date completed dd-mm-yyyy	Attempt at activity First only (F) Repeat (R) Remedial (Re)	Rating Below (B) expectations Exceeds (E) expectations	Decision of faculty Completed (C) Repeat (R) Remedial (Re)	Faculty initials	Feedback received Initial of learner
1.	Demonstrate respect for patient samples sent to the laboratory for performance of laboratory tests in the detection of microbial agents causing Infectious diseases. MI 8.11							
2.	Discuss confidentiality pertaining to patient identity in laboratory results. MI 8.12							
3.	Demonstrate confidentiality pertaining to patient identity in laboratory results. MI 8.14							

Add on Competencies as Decided by the Department of Microbiology

S. No.	Competency addressed	Name of the activity	Date completed dd-mm-yyyy	Attempt at activity First only (F) Repeat (R) Remedial (Re)	Rating Below (B) expectations Meets (M) expectations Exceeds (E) expectations or Numerical scores	Decision of faculty Completed (C) Repeat (R) Remedial (Re)	Faculty initials and date	Feedback received Initial of learner

Add on Competencies as Decided by the Department of Microbiology

S. No.	Competency addressed	Name of the activity	Date completed dd-mm-yyyy	Attempt at activity First only (F) Repeat (R) Remedial (Re)	Rating Below (B) expectations Meets (M) expectations Exceeds (E) expectations or Numerical scores	Decision of faculty Completed (C) Repeat (R) Remedial (Re)	Faculty initials and date	Feedback received Initial of learner

Add on Competencies as Decided by the Department of Microbiology

S. No.	Competency addressed	Name of the activity	Date completed dd-mm-yyyy	**Attempt at activity** First only (F) Repeat (R) Remedial (Re)	**Rating** Below (B) expectations Meets (M) expectations Exceeds (E) expectations or Numerical scores	**Decision of faculty** Completed (C) Repeat (R) Remedial (Re)	Faculty initials and date	**Feedback received** Initial of learner

Add on Competencies as Decided by the Department of Microbiology

S. No.	Competency addressed	Name of the activity	Date completed dd-mm-yyyy	Attempt at activity First only (F) Repeat (R) Remedial (Re)	Rating Below (B) expectations Meets (M) expectations Exceeds (E) expectations or Numerical scores	Decision of faculty Completed (C) Repeat (R) Remedial (Re)	Faculty initials and date	Feedback received Initial of learner

Competencies of the Procedures for Certification

S. No.	Competency addressed	Name of the activity	Number required to certify P (perform)	Date completed dd-mm-yyyy	Attempt at activity First only (F) Repeat (R) Remedial (Re)	Rating Below (B) expectations Meets (M) expectations Exceeds (E) expectations or Numerical scores	Decision of faculty Completed (C) Repeat (R) Remedial (Re)	Faculty initials and date	Feedback received Initial of learner
1.	Perform and identify the different causative agents of infectious diseases by Gram stain, ZN stain and stool routine microscopy. MI 1.2		5						
2.	Identify the common etiologic agents of upper respiratory tract infections (Gram stain). MI 6.2		3						
3.	Identify the common etiologic agents of lower respiratory tract infections (Gram stain and Acid fast stain). MI 6.3		3						
4.	Demonstrate Infection control practices and use of personal protective equipments (PPE). MI 8.7		3 each in (hand hygiene and PPE)						

Certifiable Competencies in Microbiology

Competency MI1.2

Perform and identify the different causative agents of infectious diseases by Gram stain, ZN stain and stool routine microscopy.

Specific Learning Objectives (SLOs)

1.

2.

3.

4.

Description of the Module

Reflection on Certifiable Competency

Topic 1 **Date**

Perform and identify the different causative agents of infectious diseases by Gram stain, ZN stain and stool routine microscopy.

What happened:

So what:

What next:

Signature of Teacher-in-charge

Reflection on Certifiable Competency

Topic 1 **Date**

Perform and identify the different causative agents of infectious diseases by Gram stain, ZN stain and stool routine microscopy.

What happened:

So what:

What next:

Signature of Teacher-in-charge

Note:

Certifiable Competencies in Microbiology

Competency MI6.2

Identify the common etiologic agents of upper respiratory tract infections (Gram stain).

Specific Learning Objectives (SLOs)

1.

2.

3.

4.

Description of the Module

Reflection on Certifiable Competency

Topic 2

Date

Identify the common etiologic agents of upper respiratory tract infections (Gram stain).

What happened:

So what:

What next:

Signature of Teacher-in-charge

Reflection on Certifiable Competency

Topic 2 **Date**

Identify the common etiologic agents of upper respiratory tract infections (Gram stain).

What happened:

So what:

What next:

Signature of Teacher-in-charge

Note:

Certifiable Competencies in Microbiology

Competency MI6.3

Identify the common etiologic agents of lower respiratory tract infections (Gram stain and Acid fast stain).

Specific Learning Objectives (SLOs)

1.

2.

3.

4.

Description of the Module

Reflection on Certifiable Competency

Topic 3 **Date**

Identify the common etiologic agents of lower respiratory tract infections (Gram stain and Acid fast stain).

What happened:

So what:

What next:

Signature of Teacher-in-charge

Reflection on Certifiable Competency

Topic 3 **Date**

Identify the common etiologic agents of lower respiratory tract infections (Gram stain and Acid fast stain).

What happened:

So what:

What next:

Signature of Teacher-in-charge

Note:

Certifiable Competencies in Microbiology

Competency MI8.7

Demonstrate Infection Control Practices and use of Personal Protective Equipment (PPE).

Specific Learning Objectives (SLOs)

1.

2.

3.

4.

Description of the Module

Reflection on Certifiable Competency

Topic 4

Date

Demonstrate Infection Control Practices and use of Personal Protective Equipment (PPE).

What happened:

So what:

What next:

Signature of Teacher-in-charge

Reflection on Certifiable Competency

Topic 4 **Date**

Demonstrate Infection Control Practices and use of Personal Protective Equipment (PPE).

What happened:

So what:

What next:

Signature of Teacher-in-charge

Note:

Section 2

Alignment and Integration Topics (AITOs)

Competencies of the Alignment and Integration Topics (AITOs)

S. No.	Competency addressed	Name of the activity	Number required to certify P (perform)	Date completed dd-mm-yyyy	Attempt at activity First only (F) Repeat (R) Remedial (Re)	Rating Below (B) expectations Meets (M) expectations Exceeds (E) expectations or Numerical scores	Decision of faculty Completed (C) Repeat (R) Remedial (Re)	Faculty initials and date	Feedback received Initial of learner

Competencies of the Alignment and Integration Topics (AITOs)

S. No.	Competency addressed	Name of the activity	Number required to certify P (perform)	Date completed dd-mm-yyyy	Attempt at activity First only (F) Repeat (R) Remedial (Re)	Rating Below (B) expectations Meets (M) expectations Exceeds (E) expectations or Numerical scores	Decision of faculty Completed (C) Repeat (R) Remedial (Re)	Faculty initials and date	Feedback received Initial of learner

Competencies of the Alignment and Integration Topics (AITOs)

S. No.	Competency addressed	Name of the activity	Number required to certify P (perform)	Date completed dd-mm-yyyy	Attempt at activity First only (F) Repeat (R) Remedial (Re)	Rating Below (B) expectations Meets (M) expectations Exceeds (E) expectations or Numerical scores	Decision of faculty Completed (C) Repeat (R) Remedial (Re)	Faculty initials and date	Feedback received Initial of learner

Competencies of the Alignment and Integration Topics (AITOs)

S. No.	Competency addressed	Name of the activity	Number required to certify P (perform)	Date completed dd-mm-yyyy	Attempt at activity First only (F) Repeat (R) Remedial (Re)	Rating Below (B) expectations Meets (M) expectations Exceeds (E) expectations or Numerical scores	Decision of faculty Completed (C) Repeat (R) Remedial (Re)	Faculty initials and date	Feedback received Initial of learner

Section 3 Self-directed Learning

Competencies of the Self-directed Learning

S. No.	Competency addressed	Name of the activity	Number required to certify P (perform)	Date completed dd-mm-yyyy	Attempt at activity First only (F) Repeat (R) Remedial (Re)	Rating Below (B) expectations Meets (M) expectations Exceeds (E) expectations or Numerical scores	Decision of faculty Completed (C) Repeat (R) Remedial (Re)	Faculty initials and date	Feedback received Initial of learner

Competencies of the Self-directed Learning

S. No.	Competency addressed	Name of the activity	Number required to certify P (perform)	Date completed dd-mm-yyyy	Attempt at activity First only (F) Repeat (R) Remedial (Re)	Rating Below (B) expectations Meets (M) expectations Exceeds (E) expectations or Numerical scores	Decision of faculty Completed (C) Repeat (R) Remedial (Re)	Faculty initials and date	Feedback received Initial of learner

Competencies of the Self-directed Learning

S. No.	Competency addressed	Name of the activity	Number required to certify P (perform)	Date completed dd-mm-yyyy	Attempt at activity First only (F) Repeat (R) Remedial (Re)	Rating Below (B) expectations Meets (M) expectations Exceeds (E) expectations or Numerical scores	Decision of faculty Completed (C) Repeat (R) Remedial (Re)	Faculty initials and date	Feedback received Initial of learner

Competencies of the Self-directed Learning

S. No.	Competency addressed	Name of the activity	Number required to certify P (perform)	Date completed dd-mm-yyyy	Attempt at activity First only (F) Repeat (R) Remedial (Re)	Rating Below (B) expectations Meets (M) expectations Exceeds (E) expectations or Numerical scores	Decision of faculty Completed (C) Repeat (R) Remedial (Re)	Faculty initials and date	Feedback received Initial of learner

Self-directed Learning (Seminars, Projects, Quizzes)

S. No.	Date	Topic learnt	Mode of bearing (project/quiz/seminar)	Signature of teacher
1.				
2.				
3.				
4.				
5.				
6.				
7.				
8.				
9.				
10.				

* *Total allotted SDL hours for microbiology is 10 hours*

Self-directed Learning (Seminars, Projects, Quizzes)

S. No.	Date	Topic learnt	Mode of bearing (project/quiz/seminar)	Signature of teacher
11.				
12.				
13.				
14.				
15.				
16.				
17.				
18.				
19.				
20.				

* ***Total allotted SDL hours for microbiology is 10 hours***

Reflection on Self-directed Learning

Topic: **Date:**

What happened:

So what:

What next:

Signature of Teacher-in-charge

Topic: **Date:**

What happened:

So what:

What next:

Signature of Teacher-in-charge

Reflection on Self-directed Learning

Topic: **Date:**

What happened:

So what:

What next:

Signature of Teacher-in-charge

Topic: **Date:**

What happened:

So what:

What next:

Signature of Teacher-in-charge

Reflection on Self-directed Learning

Topic: **Date:**

What happened:

So what:

What next:

Signature of Teacher-in-charge

Topic: **Date:**

What happened:

So what:

What next:

Signature of Teacher-in-charge

Reflection on Self-directed Learning

Topic: **Date:**

What happened:

So what:

What next:

Signature of Teacher-in-charge

Topic: **Date:**

What happened:

So what:

What next:

Signature of Teacher-in-charge

Reflection on Self-directed Learning

Topic: **Date:**

What happened:

So what:

What next:

Signature of Teacher-in-charge

Topic: **Date:**

What happened:

So what:

What next:

Signature of Teacher-in-charge

Reflection on Self-directed Learning

Topic: **Date:**

What happened:

So what:

What next:

Signature of Teacher-in-charge

Topic: **Date:**

What happened:

So what:

What next:

Signature of Teacher-in-charge

Reflection on Self-directed Learning

Topic: **Date:**

What happened:

So what:

What next:

Signature of Teacher-in-charge

Topic: **Date:**

What happened:

So what:

What next:

Signature of Teacher-in-charge

Reflection on Self-directed Learning

Topic: **Date:**

What happened:

So what:

What next:

Signature of Teacher-in-charge

Topic: **Date:**

What happened:

So what:

What next:

Signature of Teacher-in-charge

Reflection on Self-directed Learning

Topic: **Date:**

What happened:

So what:

What next:

Signature of Teacher-in-charge

Topic: **Date:**

What happened:

So what:

What next:

Signature of Teacher-in-charge

Reflection on Self-directed Learning

Topic: **Date:**

What happened:

So what:

What next:

Signature of Teacher-in-charge

Topic: **Date:**

What happened:

So what:

What next:

Signature of Teacher-in-charge

Section 4 Pandemic Management

Pandemic Management Modules for 1st and 2nd Professional MBBS taken up by Microbiology Department

S. No.	Competency addressed	Name of the activity	Date completed dd-mm-yyyy	Attempt at activity First only (F) Repeat (R) Remedial (Re)	Rating Below (B) expectations Meets (M) expectations Exceeds (E) expectations or Numerical scores	Decision of faculty Completed (C) Repeat (R) Remedial (Re)	Faculty initials and date	Feedback received Initial of learner
PHASE - I								
1.	Infection control: Part - I Infection control practices— hand washing, decontamination use of PPEs. Module 1.1							
PHASE - II								
2.	Infection control: Part II Airborne precautions, contact precautions, infection control committee. Module 2.1							
3.	Sample collection, microbial diagnosis, serologic tests and their performance parameters. Module 2.3							

Pandemic Management Module for Phase - I MBBS

Module PM 1.1: Infection Control Practices–Part I

Background

Exposure to infectious organisms is a common phenomenon but development of disease following such exposures can be easily prevented by following certain practices that have been labeled as "standard precautions". It has been shown in studies that students who receive education about standard precautions have a higher level of knowledge and comply better. Various studies along with "patient safety module" by WHO strongly recommends incorporation of infection control modules in the curriculum of medical schools as medical students, the future doctors need to understand these concepts at an early stage to be able to incorporate them in their practice. The student must be taught scientific bases of these practices that can protect against infections both in community as well as hospital settings. The student should be taught about the basics of infection control practices with emphasis on ability to use personal protective equipment (PPE) optimally.

This module is aimed at enabling the learner to practise standard infection control practices including proper and consistent hand washing, use of PPEs and to familiarize with various disinfection and antiseptic procedures.

Competencies Addressed

The student should be able to:	Level	Major department(s) to coordinate
1. Demonstrate proper hand washing	SH	Microbiology
2. Demonstrate donning and doffing of PPE	SH	

Learning Experience

Year of study: Professional year 1

Hours: 4 hours

1. Interactive discussion - 1 hour
   a. Basics of infection and chain of transmission
   b. Significance and ways of infection prevention
   c. Role of hand in spread of infections and importance of hand hygiene in prevention of spread of infections
   d. Components of standard precautions and use of PPE
   e. Cough etiquette.
2. DOAP session on hand washing, use of gloves, mask, donning and doffing of PPE - 1 hour
3. Visit to the hospital and discussion with the staff about the infection control practices followed by them - 1 hour
4. Debriefing and feedback - 1 hour.

Assessment

- **Formative:** Viva can be used. This could be done immediately after the module and/or later with internal assessment. The technique of hand washing and donning an doffing of gloves can be randomly observed during conduct of practical sessions in first MBBS particularly in dissection halls. Peer feedback can also be incorporated.
- **Summative:** Not required.

Resources

https://www.cdc.gov/infectioncontrol/training/infection-control.html.

Module PM 1.1: Infection Control Practices - I

What happened:

So what:

What next

Date: **Signature of Teacher-in-charge**

Module PM 1.1: Infection Control Practices - I

What happened:

So what:

What next:

Date: **Signature of Teacher-in-charge**

Note:

Note:

Pandemic Management Module for Phase - II MBBS

Module PM 2.1: Infection Control Practices–Part II

Background

The basics of infection and components of the standard precaution have been covered in the first phase. The second phase student is better equipped to understand the details of transmission-based precautions as they now learn about the microbes along with disinfection and antiseptic procedures in detail. This is also the right time to introduce a student to the roles and responsibilities of an infection control team in a hospital.

This module is aimed at enabling the learner to identify the most probable route of spread of a particular microbe causing infection and based upon that, identify which transmission-based precaution need to be adhered to along with standard infection control practices.

Competencies Addressed

The student should be able to:	Level	Major department(s) to coordinate
1. Describe and discuss the implementation of airborne and contact precautions in a specific clinical situation	KH	Microbiology
2. Describe and discuss the functioning of institutional Infection Control Committee	KH	

Learning Experience

Year of study: Professional year 2

Hours: 4 hours

1. Interactive discussion - 1 hour
   a. Revisit the various routes of spread of infections
   b. Need for isolation of patients in various circumstances
   c. Airborne and contact precautions including use of PPEs
   d. Disinfection and antisepsis in patient care
   e. Roles and responsibilities of infection control team.
2. Small group case discussion followed by plenary - 1.5 hours.

   Example of case study

   Rajani, 34 years has returned home from Italy, at a time when that country is having an epidemic of a new virus infection. She has mild cough and sore throat. When she develops severe breathlessness, she is admitted in the general ward of the hospital. You have been asked to take a detailed history and examine the patient.
   - What precautions are necessary in this case?
   - What precautions are advised for the subordinate staff attending her?
3. Visit to the isolation ward in the hospital with discussion with the staff about the precautions they take - 1 hour
4. Debriefing and feedback - 0.5 hour.

Assessment

- **Formative:** OSCE, Viva, MCQs can be used.
- **Summative:** OSCE, Viva, MCQs.

Resources

- https://www.who.int/diseasecontrol_emergencies/training/m4_infection.pdf?ua=1
- https://www.cdc.gov/infectioncontrol/training/infection-control.html.

Module PM 2.1: Infection Control Practices - II

What happened:

So what:

What next:

Date: **Signature of Teacher-in-charge**

Module PM 2.1: Infection Control Practices - II

What happened:

So what:

What next:

Date: **Signature of Teacher-in-charge**

Note:

Note:

Module PM 2.3: Diagnostic Tools

Background

Diagnostics are a fundamental component of successful outbreak containment or control strategies, being involved at every stage of an outbreak, from initial detection to eventual resolution. Each individual pathogen presents specific diagnostic challenges.

Pandemics are caused by either emergence or re-emergence of microbes. In case of re-emergence, availability of validated diagnostic protocols and tools make laboratory confirmation of the cases easy but this is not the case when we have newly evolved microbes causing pandemic. The laboratory diagnostic tests are either not available and if available, they need to be validated and their performance characteristics like sensitivity, specificity, positive predictive and negative predictive value studied before they can be used for diagnosis. The healthcare professionals are faced with various dilemmas at these times which can range from a very basic query like the best time and best sample that needs to be collected, to sensitivity and specificity of a chosen procedure that can be isolation of microbes, antigen or antibody detection or gene that needs to be detected in molecular diagnostics.

Thus, the questions are innumerable and it becomes important to train a medical student to deal with such dilemmas in the diagnosis of an infection particularly during pandemics. They must be taught to choose and collect the most appropriate clinical sample in a suitable container with/without transport media, at the most appropriate time from a suspected case during pandemic and interpret the results of the test keeping in mind various performance characteristics and validation requirements.

Competencies Addressed

The student should be able to:	Level	Major department(s) to coordinate
1. Describe specimen selection, collection, transportation and storage requirement during a pandemic	KH	Microbiology
2. Choose and collect the most appropriate clinical sample in a suitable container at the most appropriate time from a suspected case during pandemic (or in a simulated environment)	SH	
3. Demonstrate appropriate safety measures in handling and processing of clinical specimens (use of PPE, etc.)	SH	
4. Discuss various diagnostic modalities available for an infectious disease. Explain sensitivity, specificity, positive predictive value and negative predictive value of each of the diagnostic test/modality	KH	
5. Chose the most appropriate diagnostic test keeping in mind sensitivity, specificity, positive and negative predictive value of the diagnostic test/modality available	SH	

Learning Experience

Year of study: Professional year 2

Hours: 6 hours

1. Exploratory and interactive theory session - 1 hour
2. Sample collection demo and hand on in skill lab - 1 hour
3. Visit to laboratory with demonstration of diagnostic test - 1 hour
4. Small group activity, where students can be asked to discuss different test reports of suspected cases with performance characteristic and asked to interpret followed by discussion on choosing a lab test - 2 hours
5. Discussion and closure -1 hour.

Assessment

- **Formative:** Required by assignments, OSPE, Viva.
- **Summative:** Required by OSPE, SAQ, MCQ.

Resources

- Kelly-Cirino CD, Nkengasong J, Kettler H, et al. Importance of diagnostics in epidemic and pandemic preparedness. BMJ Global Health 2019;4: e001179.
- Miller JM, Binnicker MJ, Campbell S, Carroll KC, Chapin KC, Gilligan PH, et al A Guide to Utilization of the Microbiology Laboratory for Diagnosis of Infectious Diseases: 2018. Update by the Infectious Diseases Society of America and the American Society for Microbiology. Clinical Infectious Diseases. 2018 67(6):e1-e94.
- Washington JA. Principles of Diagnosis. In: Baron S (ed.). Medical Microbiology. 4th edition. Galveston (TX): University of Texas Medical Branch at Galveston; 1996. Chapter 10. Available from: https://www.ncbi.nlm.nih. gov/ books/NBK8014/.

Module PM 2.3: Diagnostic Tools

What happened:

So what:

What next:

Date: **Signature of Teacher-in-charge**

Module PM 2.3: Diagnostic Tools

What happened:

So what:

What next:

Date: **Signature of Teacher-in-charge**

Note:

Note:

Section 5

AETCOM

AETCOM Modules for 2nd Professional MBBS taken up by Microbiology Department

S. No.	Competency addressed	Name of the activity	Date completed dd-mm-yyyy	Attempt at activity First only (F) Repeat (R) Remedial (Re)	Rating Below (B) expectations Meets (M) expectations Exceeds (E) expectations or Numerical scores	Decision of faculty Completed (C) Repeat (R) Remedial (Re)	Faculty initials and date	Feedback received Initial of learner
1.	The foundations of communication – 2. Module 2.1							
2.	The foundations of bioethics. Module 2.2							
3.	Health care as a right. Module 2.3							
4.	Working in a healthcare team. Module 2.4							
5.	Bioethics continued —case studies on patient autonomy and decision making. Module 2.5							
6.	Bioethics continued – case studies on autonomy and decision making. Module 2.6							
7.	Bioethics continued —case studies on autonomy and decision making. Module 2.7							
8.	What does it mean to be family member of a sick patient? Module 2.8							

Note: Distribution of topics amongst the departments should be finalized by the concerned departments only.

Module 2.1: The Foundations of Communication - 2

Background

Communication is a fundamental prerequisite of the medical profession and beside skills is crucial in ensuring professional success for doctors. This module continues to provide an emphasis on effective communication skills. During professional year II, the emphasis is on active listening and data gathering.

Competencies Addressed

The student should be able to:	Level
1. Demonstrate ability to communicate to patients in a patient, respectful, non-threatening, non- judgmental and empathetic manner	SH

Learning Experience

Year of study: Professional year 2

Hours: 5 (1 + 2 + 1 + 1)

i. Introductory small group session - 1 hour
ii. Focused small group session - 2 hours
iii. Skills lab session – 1 hour
iv. Discussion and closure of case - 1 hour

Contents

1. Introductory small group session on the principles of communication with focus on opening the discussion, listening and gathering data.
2. Focused small group session with role play or videos where the students have an opportunity to observe, criticize and discuss common mistakes in opening the discussion, listening and data gathering.
3. Skills lab sessions where students can perform tasks on standardized or regular patients with opportunity for self-critique, critique by patient and by the facilitator.

Assessment

1. **Formative:** Participation in session 2 and performance in session 3 may be used as part of formative assessment.
2. **Summative:** May be deferred.

Resources

1. Makoul G. Essential elements of communication in medical encounters: The Kalamazoo consensus statement. Acad Med. 2001;76(4): 390-3.
2. Hausberg M. Enhancing medical students' communication skills: Development and evaluation of an undergraduate training program. BMC Medical Education. 2012; 12:16.

Module 2.1: The Foundations of Communication - 2

What happened:

So what:

What next:

Date: **Signature of Teacher-in-charge**

Module 2.1: The Foundations of Communication - 2

What happened:

So what:

What next:

Date: **Signature of Teacher-in-charge**

Note:

Note:

Module 2.2: The Foundations of Bioethics

Background

An introductory session in a large group that provides an overview of the evolution and the fundamental principles of bioethics including the cardinal pillars of ethics viz., autonomy, beneficence, nonmaleficence and justice.

Competencies Addressed

The student should be able to:	Level
1. Describe and discuss the role of nonmaleficence as a guiding principle in patient care	KH
2. Describe and discuss the role of autonomy and shared responsibility as a guiding principle in patient care	KH
3. Describe and discuss the role of beneficence of a guiding principle in patient care	KH
4. Describe and discuss the role of a physician in health care system	KH
5. Describe and discuss the role of justice as a guiding principle in patient care	KH

Learning Experience

Year of study: Professional year 2

Hours: 2 large group session - 2 hours

Contents

This module is a large group learning session that can be made interactive by illustrative examples.

Assessment

Summative: Short notes on: (a) autonomy, (b) beneficence, (c) nonmaleficence.

Resources

A review of the four principles of bioethics is found here: ttp://archive.journalchirohumanities.com/Vol%2014/JChiroprHumanit 2007 v14_34-40.pdf

Module 2.2: The Foundations of Bioethics

What happened:

So what:

What next:

Date: **Signature of Teacher-in-charge**

Module 2.2: The Foundations of Bioethics

What happened:

So what:

What next:

Date: **Signature of Teacher-in-charge**

Note:

Note:

Module 2.3: Health Care as a Right

Background

This session is aimed at introducing students to healthcare systems, their access, equity in access, the impact of socio-economic situations in determining healthcare access and the role of doctors as key players in the healthcare system.

Competencies Addressed

The student should be able to:	Level
1. Describe and discuss the role of nonmaleficence as a guiding principle in patient care	KH

Learning Experience

Year of study: Professional year 2

Hours: 2

i. Participatory student seminar - 2 hours

Contents

This module may be done as a participatory student seminar with debates on the more controversial issues to increase a reflective process.

Focus may be on:

1. Is health care a right?
2. What are the implications of health care as a right?
3. What are the social and economic implications of health care as a right?
4. What are the missing links? (see resource 2 for a brief overview)
5. What are the implications for doctors?

Assessment

Summative: Short note on barriers to implementation of health care as a universal right

Resources

1. The Universal Declaration of Human Rights. http://www.un.org/en/documents/udhr/
2. Missing links in universal health care. http://www.thehindu.com/opinion/lead/missing-links-in-universal-health-care/article6618667.ece

Module 2.3: Health Care as a Right

What happened:

So what:

What next:

Date: **Signature of Teacher-in-charge**

Module 2.3: Health Care as a Right

What happened:

So what:

What next:

Date:

Signature of Teacher-in-charge

Note:

Note:

Module 2.4: Working in a Healthcare Team

Background

This session is aimed at introducing students to healthcare systems and their functioning. It allows students to "tag along" with members of healthcare teams, observe their work and gain experience about their perspectives. It is hoped that this experience will help students to understand the need for collaborative work in health care, how each member of the healthcare team is important and also develop respect.

Competencies Addressed

The student should be able to:	Level
1. Demonstrate ability to work in a team of peers and superiors.	SH
2. Demonstrate respect in relationship with patients, fellow team members, superiors and other health care workers.	SH

Learning Experience

Year of study: Professional year 2

Hours: 6 hours (4 hours "tag along" + 2 hours discussion)

i. "Tag along" session in hospital - 2 × 2 hours
ii. Small group discussion session - 2 hours

Contents

This module may be done as two interdependent sessions:

1. A "tag along" session where students spend time with other healthcare workers including nurses, technicians and others, observe their work, their interactions, conduct a small interview with them and write a narrative based on this interview.
2. A small group discussion which is based on the students' observations, experiences, reflections and inferences and what must be done by them to work as an integral part of the healthcare team.

Assessment

Formative: Student participation in session 2 with assessment of submitted narrative.

Module 2.4: Working in a Healthcare Team

What happened:

So what:

What next:

Date: **Signature of Teacher-in-charge**

Module 2.4: Working in a Healthcare Team

What happened:

So what:

What next:

Date: **Signature of Teacher-in-charge**

Note:

Note:

Module 2.5: Bioethics Continued—
Case Studies on Patient Autonomy and Decision-making

Background

The important parts of ethical care of the patient are best learnt in a hybrid problem-based format with additional lectures and other sessions that allow students to learn collaboratively with different learning styles. A guide for case discussion is provided in the resources section of this module and may be used as a guide for other modules. The key element is that students remain in the same group with the same facilitator since groups mature in their learning over time.

Competencies Addressed

The student should be able to:	Level
1. Identify, discuss and defend medicolegal, sociocultural and ethical issues as it pertains to patient autonomy, patient rights and shared responsibility in health care.	KH

Learning Experience

Year of study: Professional year 2

Hours: 6 hours

i. Introduction and group formation - 1 hour
ii. Case introduction - 1 hour
iii. Self-directed learning - 2 hours
iv. Anchoring lecture - 1 hour
v. Case resolution - 1 hour

Case: The Cover Up

You evaluate Mrs Lakshmi Srinivasan who is a 48-year-old woman presenting with lymphadenopathy. She had been complaining of mild fever and weight loss for the past 4–5 months. Examination of the neck shows large rubbery lymph nodes that are present also in the axilla and the groin. There is a palpable spleen. She is accompanied by her caring husband.

Lakshmi undergoes a lymph node biopsy and the pathologist calls you and tells you that she has a lymphoma. That evening Mr Srinivasan comes in first into your office and leaves the report on your table. As you read the description you realize that the final diagnosis has been altered to tuberculosis by whitening out the pathologist's report. When you look up he tells you "Sir, I googled lymphoma—it is almost like a cancer. My wife cannot handle that diagnosis. She has always been a worried frightened person. I want you to tell my wife that she had TB. She is waiting outside, doctor. I thought I will call her in after I had a chat about this with you".

Points for Discussion

1. Does the patient have a right to know their diagnosis?
2. What should the patient be told about their diagnosis, therapy and prognosis?
3. How much should be told to a patient about their illness?
4. Are there exceptions to full disclosure? Can family members request withholding of information from patient?

Assessment

1. **Formative:** The student may be assessed based on their active participation in the sessions.
2. **Summative:** Short questions on: (1) Define patient autonomy, (2) Contrast autonomy and paternalism, (3) What are the responsibilities of patients and doctors in shared decision making? (4) What is full and reasonable disclosure?

   The suggested location, duration and requirements are as in item 2.

   Once the case (or part of the case) is resolved, the next case (or the next part of the case) is introduced.

Module 2.5: Bioethics Continued— Case Studies on Patient Autonomy and Decision-making

What happened:

So what:

What next:

Date: **Signature of Teacher-in-charge**

Module 2.5: Bioethics Continued— Case Studies on Patient Autonomy and Decision-making

What happened:

So what:

What next:

Date:

Signature of Teacher-in-charge

Note:

Note:

Module 2.6: Bioethics Continued—Case Studies on Autonomy and Decision-making

Background

This introduces the student to further issues in autonomy including competence and capacity to make decisions (also *see* Module 2.5).

Competencies Addressed

The student should be able to:	Level
1. Identify, discuss and defend medicolegal, sociocultural and ethical issues as they pertain to refusal of care including do not resuscitate and withdrawal of life support	KH

Learning Experience

Year of study: Professional year 2

Hours: 5

i. Introduction of case - 1 hour
ii. Self-directed learning - 2 hours
iii. Anchoring lecture - 1 hour
iv. Discussion and closure of case - 1 hour

Case: Life on a Machine

You are taking care of 78-year-old Mrs Mythili who was living all alone in an apartment with only a live-in caretaker, 3 streets away from your clinic. She is a widow and her only son emigrated to the US 32 years ago. He visits her once a year. One year ago, she had a fall with a hip fracture that healed badly. She has hypertension which is reasonably controlled on medications. She continues to come to your clinic once a month. Four months ago, she spent some time talking about her sister who recently died following metastatic breast cancer. "My sister suffered a lot, doctor - they put a tube down her throat to breathe. Even when her heart stopped they kept thumping her chest - it was awful. If I ever fall sick I don't want to go through all this. Promise me, doctor, that you won't do all of this to me. I have lived all alone since my husband died but I have lived independently - now I don't want to depend on a machine to live". You had reassured her that she would be ok and this was just the recent death of her sister affecting her. On subsequent visits she would still bring up this issue and state that there was no use of her living as a burden to anyone and that no one should endure what her sister had undergone.

One day you get a call from the Emergency Room of the local hospital stating that Mrs Mythili has been admitted by the caretaker. She had developed fever and shortness of breath. She was brought hypoxic to the emergency room and they had intubated her. Chest X-ray revealed a large pneumonic patch. Laboratory testing revealed hyponatremia. When you visited her she is somewhat drowsy, intubated and restrained. The nurse tells you that she is sometimes lucid; at other times not even able to recognize her son who was there since this morning. She points out at the ET and makes a pleading gesture to remove it. Her son accosts you in the hallway. He tells you that he got a call while he was traveling in Singapore and took the first flight out to be with his mom. He was very distressed at his mother's health and that he wants "everything" possible done for her. You ask him if she had ever indicated what she wanted to be done if she were to require hospitalization and intubation—he says that he used to speak to her every month on the phone and she was always cheerful and enquiring about her grandchildren but did not talk about her health.

Points for Discussion

1. Extent of patient autonomy
2. Elements in decision-making: Competency vs. capacity
3. Surrogacy in decision making
4. Autonomy vs. beneficence
5. How much does family wishes count?
6. Legal, ethical and social aspects of 'Do not resuscitate'.

Assessment

1. **Formative:** The student may be assessed based on their active participation in the sessions.
2. **Summative:** Short questions on: (a) What determines decision-making capacity and competency? (b) Who has the right to make decisions for a patient who cannot determine for himself?

Resources

See Module 2.5.

Module 2.6: Bioethics Continued—Case Studies on Autonomy and Decision-making

What happened:

So what:

What next:

Date: **Signature of Teacher-in-charge**

Module 2.6: Bioethics Continued—Case Studies on Autonomy and Decision-making

What happened:

So what:

What next:

Date: **Signature of Teacher-in-charge**

Note:

Note:

Module 2.7: Bioethics Continued—Case Studies on Autonomy and Decision-making

Background

This introduces the student to further issues in autonomy including informed consent and refusal (also *see* module 2.5).

Competencies Addressed

The student should be able to:	Level
1. Identify, discuss and defend, medicolegal, sociocultural and ethical issues as they pertain to consent for surgical procedures.	KH

Learning Experience

Year of study: Professional year 2

Hours: 5

i. Introduction of case - 1 hour
ii. Self-directed learning - 2 hours
iii. Anchoring lecture - 1 hour
iv. Discussion and closure of case - 1 hour

Case: Who is the Doctor?

A 54-year-old man named Mr Surendra Patel is admitted for acute chest pain in a medical centre. His father had died of a myocardial infarction at the age of 60. Two years ago, his brother had been admitted to a hospital with a myocardial infarction and had died after complications following an angioplasty. Mr Patel is a diabetic and is on multiple oral hypoglycemic agents with moderate control. He is a businessman with his own small industry. After initial stabilization, the patient is comfortable and pain-free after analgesics, nitrates and statins. Preliminary blood tests and ECG confirm an acute coronary event. The next morning, the senior cardiologist makes rounds and reviews the patient. "You have unstable angina, Mr Patel and require an angiogram. You may also require either a stent or coronary bypass after the procedure. The nurse will provide you with the necessary paperwork. Please sign it and I will plan the procedure for 4.35 am tomorrow morning." "Doctor sahib", asked Mr Patel, "I am not comfortable with the idea of an angiogram; my brother died on the table when an angioplasty was being done. Aren't there other tests that you can do? I am not happy with this option". "Your brother would have had it with someone else, Mr Patel - I have the best hands in town; nothing will happen when I do it" retorted the cardiologist. "But aren't there any other options to see what I have? Is this the only test? I have read somewhere that you can do a CT angiogram", persisted Mr Patel. "Are you the doctor or am I the doctor?" retorted the cardiologist angrily. "If you are ready to do as I say, sign the papers and I will see you in the Cath lab tomorrow. Otherwise you are free to get discharged". He stomped out.

Points for Discussion

1. Extent of patient autonomy.
2. Informed consent and informed refusal.
3. Conflict between autonomy and beneficence.
4. What should the patient be told about a procedure?
5. What must the informed consent include?

Assessment

1. **Formative:** The student may be assessed based on their active participation in the sessions.
2. **Summative:** Short questions on: (1) What is informed consent? (2) What is informed refusal?

Resources

See Module 2.5.

Module 2.7: Bioethics Continued—Case Studies on Autonomy and Decision-making

What happened:

So what:

What next:

Date: **Signature of Teacher-in-charge**

Module 2.7: Bioethics Continued—Case Studies on Autonomy and Decision-making

What happened:

So what:

What next:

Date:

Signature of Teacher-in-charge

Note:

Note:

Module 2.8: What Does it Mean to be Family Member of a Sick Patient?

Background

Doctors deal with human suffering throughout their professional careers. A balanced approach to the patient care experience requires an understanding of support systems of patients, priorities coping and emotions of families, the role of the doctor, an exploration of empathy vs. equanimity and the difference between healing and curing and support.

Competencies Addressed

The student should be able to:	Level
1. Demonstrate empathy in patient encounters.	SH

Learning Experience

Year of study: Professional year 2

Hours: 6 (includes 2 hours of SDL)

i. Hospital visit and interviews - 2 hours
ii. Large group discussions with patients' relatives - 1 hour
iii. Self-directed learning - 2 hours
iv. Discussion and closure - 1 hour

1. Students are assigned to patients in the hospital, interview their family about their illnesses, experience, reactions, emotions, outlook and expectations (or can be done in a controlled environment with standardized patients).
2. Family members of patients with different illnesses may be brought to a large group discussion with permission and an interactive discussion (based on the items outlined in option 1. Can use standardized patients)
3. Self-directed learning where students write a report from reflection based on sessions 1 and 2 and on other readings, TV series, movies, etc.
4. A closure session with students to share their reflections based on 1, 2 and 3 so that it includes how they intend to incorporate the lessons learnt in patient care.

Assessment

1. **Formative:** The student may be assessed based on their active participation in the sessions and submission of the written narrative.
2. **Summative:** Short questions on the role of doctors in the community and expectations of society form doctors, e.g. What is empathy? What is the role of empathy in the care of patients?

Module 2.8: What Does it Mean to be Family Member of a Sick Patient?

What happened:

So what:

What next:

Date: **Signature of Teacher-in-charge**

Module 2.8: What Does it Mean to be Family Member of a Sick Patient?

What happened:

So what:

What next:

Date: **Signature of Teacher-in-charge**

Note:

Note:

Section 6

Humanities

Competencies Related to Humanities

S. No.	**Competency addressed**	**Name of the activity**	**Date completed dd-mm-yyyy**	**Attempt at activity** First only (F) Repeat (R) Remedial (Re)	**Rating** Below (B) expectations Meets (M) expectations Exceeds (E) expectations or Numerical scores	**Decision of faculty** Completed (C) Repeat (R) Remedial (Re)	**Faculty initials and date**	**Feedback received** Initial of learner

S. No.	Competency addressed	Name of the activity	Date completed dd-mm-yyyy	Attempt at activity First only (F) Repeat (R) Remedial (Re)	Rating Below (B) expectations Meets (M) expectations Exceeds (E) expectations or Numerical scores	Decision of faculty Completed (C) Repeat (R) Remedial (Re)	Faculty initials and date	Feedback received Initial of learner

Note:

Section 7

Sports/Physical Education

Competencies Related to Sports/Physical Education

S. No.	Competency addressed	Name of the activity	Date completed dd-mm-yyyy	Attempt at activity First only (F) Repeat (R) Remedial (Re)	Rating Below (B) expectations Meets (M) expectations Exceeds (E) expectations or Numerical scores	Decision of faculty Completed (C) Repeat (R) Remedial (Re)	Faculty initials and date	Feedback received Initial of learner

S. No.	Competency addressed	Name of the activity	Date completed dd-mm-yyyy	Attempt at activity First only (F) Repeat (R) Remedial (Re)	Rating Below (B) expectations Meets (M) expectations Exceeds (E) expectations or Numerical scores	Decision of faculty Completed (C) Repeat (R) Remedial (Re)	Faculty initials and date	Feedback received Initial of learner

Note:

Section 8 Extracurricular Activities

Competencies Related to Extracurricular Activities

S. No.	Competency addressed	Name of the activity	Date completed dd-mm-yyyy	**Attempt at activity** First only (F) Repeat (R) Remedial (Re)	**Rating** Below (B) expectations Meets (M) expectations Exceeds (E) expectations or Numerical scores	**Decision of faculty** Completed (C) Repeat (R) Remedial (Re)	Faculty initials and date	**Feedback received** Initial of learner

S. No.	Competency addressed	Name of the activity	Date completed dd-mm-yyyy	Attempt at activity First only (F) Repeat (R) Remedial (Re)	Rating Below (B) expectations Meets (M) expectations Exceeds (E) expectations or Numerical scores	Decision of faculty Completed (C) Repeat (R) Remedial (Re)	Faculty initials and date	Feedback received Initial of learner

Note:

Section 9 Attendance Records

Attendance Record of the Student

Roll No........................................ **MBBS Batch**................................... **University Reg. No.** ....

Name... **College Name**...

S. No.	Term	Subject	Theory (%)	Practical (%)	Signature of student	Signature of teacher
1.	I Term	Microbiology				
2.	II Term					
3.	Overall attendance					

Note: Above information is for the benefit of students and parents. In case of any discrepancy departmental record will be treated as final.

Instructions as per NMC: Attendance requirements are 75% in theory and 80% in practical/clinical for eligibility to appear for the examinations in that subject. In subjects that are taught in more than one phase—the learner must have 75% attendance in theory and 80% in practical in each phase of instruction in that subject.

(Professor and Head)
Department of Microbiology
.... **Medical College**

Details of Attending Extra Classes
[For Poor Attendance (If Any)]

Roll No....................................... **MBBS Batch**.................................... **University Reg. No.** ....

Name.. **College Name**...

S. No.	Date	Topics	Signature of student	Signature of teacher
		Total hours =		

Note: Above information is for the benefit of students and parents. In case of any discrepancy departmental record will be treated as final.

(Professor and Head)
Department of Microbiology
.... **Medical College**

Section 10

Records of Internal Assessment

Final Records of Internal Assessment Examinations

Roll No........................................ **MBBS Batch**.................................. **University Reg. No.** ....

Name.. **College Name**...

S. No.	Term	Subject	Theory exam	Practical exam	Signature of student	Signature of HOD
1.	I Terminal assessment	Microbiology	/100	/100		
2.	II Terminal assessment		/100	/100		
3.	III Terminal (Pre-university) assessment		/200	/100		
4.	Betterment examinations (If any)		/200	/100		
5.	Final internal assessment		/100	/100		

Note:

- **IA:** 50% combined in theory and practical (not less than 40% in each) for eligibility for appearing in university examinations.
- **University examinations:** Mandatory 50% marks in each theory and practical examination separately. [Practical = Practical/Clinical + Viva] [Theory = Theory paper(s) only]

Section 11

Final Summary

S. No.	Description	Date		Status
		From	To	Complete/incomplete
1.	Microbiology Logbook			
2.	Alignment and Integration Topics (AITOs)			
3.	AETCOM			
4.	Humanities			
5.	Sports/Physical Education			
6.	Extracurricular Activities			

Note: Minimum allotted time for sports and extracurricular activities are 28 hours.

(Professor and Head)
Department of Microbiology
.... **Medical College**